High Calories Recipes for Weight Gain

By

Clark Owens

Table of contents

Introduction

Gaining weight can be just as challenging as losing it, especially for those looking to add healthy pounds or muscle mass. For individuals aiming to increase their calorie intake in a nutritious and deliberate manner, high-calorie recipes play a pivotal role. These recipes aren't solely about consuming any food available in large quantities; they
focus on a balanced approach that incorporates nutrient-dense ingredients to promote weight gain in a healthy way.

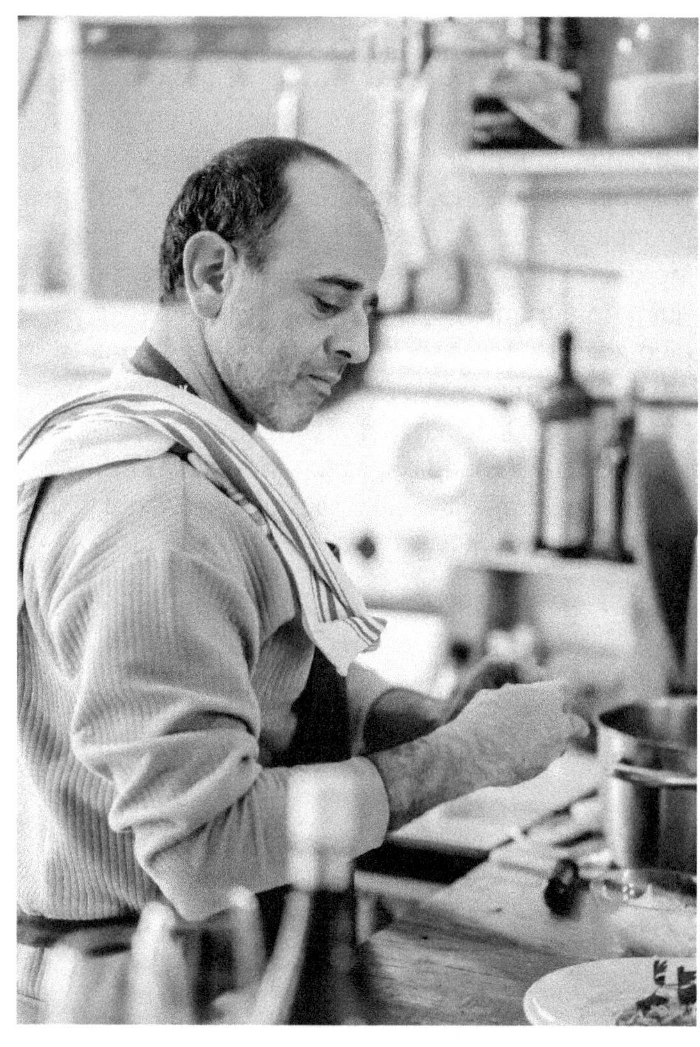

Understanding Weight Gain and Nutrition

Before delving into high-calorie recipes, it's essential to understand the principles behind healthy weight gain. Simply
Increasing calorie intake without considering nutritional value can lead to an imbalance in one's diet. Optimal weight gain involves a blend of macronutrients (carbohydrates, proteins, and fats) and micronutrients (vitamins and minerals). High-calorie recipes crafted for weight gain purposefully combine these elements to ensure a well-rounded approach.

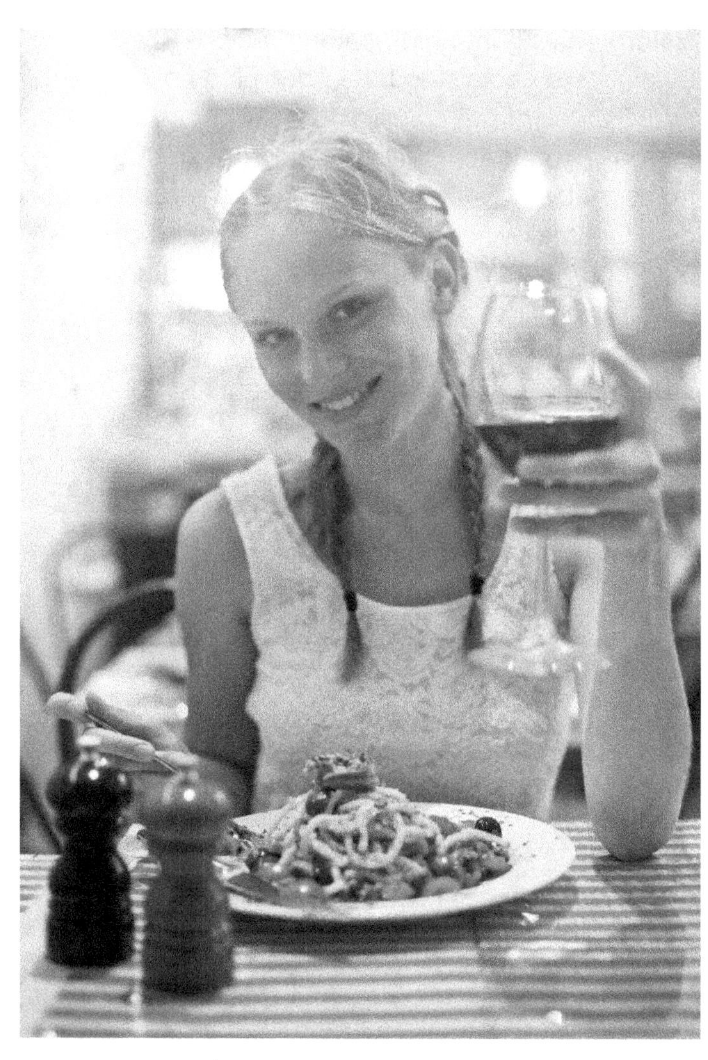

Balanced Macronutrient Composition

Carbohydrates serve as the body's primary energy source, making them a fundamental component of high-calorie recipes. However, focusing solely on carbs might lead to gaining weight in an unhealthy manner. Hence, the inclusion of proteins and healthy fats becomes crucial. Proteins aid in muscle repair and growth, contributing to overall body strength. Healthy fats, such as those found in avocados, nuts, and seeds, not only add calories but also provide essential nutrients, aiding in bodily functions.

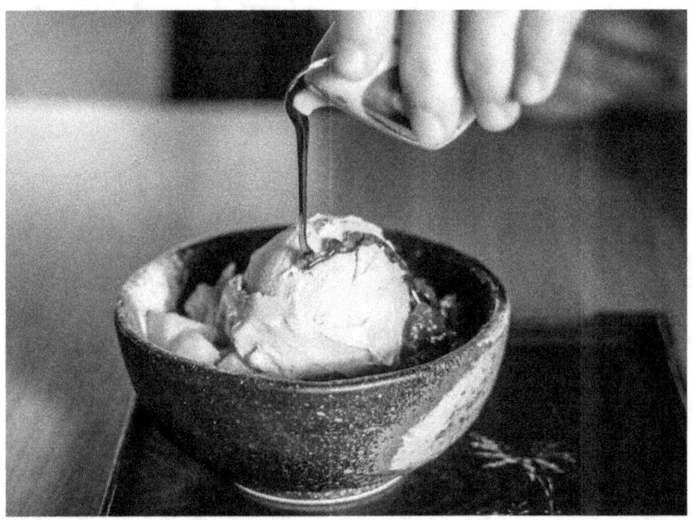

The Importance of Nutrient Density

High-calorie recipes for weight gain emphasise nutrient-dense ingredients. While the goal is to increase calorie intake, it's equally crucial to ensure these calories come from wholesome sources. Ingredients rich in vitamins, minerals, and antioxidants support overall health while promoting weight gain. Leafy greens, colourful fruits, lean proteins, and whole grains form the backbone of these recipes, offering a wealth of nutrients alongside the necessary calories.

Customization and Adaptation

The beauty of high-calorie recipes lies in their adaptability to individual preferences and dietary needs. Whether someone prefers a vegetarian, vegan, or omnivorous diet, these recipes can be tailored accordingly.
Additionally, they can be adjusted for those with specific dietary requirements or allergies, ensuring a wide range of individuals can benefit from them.

Practicality and Accessibility

These recipes aren't overly complicated or inaccessible. They are designed to be practical for everyday cooking, considering the time constraints many people face. Simplicity in preparation doesn't compromise their nutritional value or taste. By using readily available ingredients and straightforward cooking methods, these recipes become approachable for anyone seeking to enhance their calorie intake.

Conclusion

High-calorie recipes for weight gain offer a structured approach towards healthy and intentional weight increase. By balancing macronutrients, emphasising nutrient density, and allowing for customization, these recipes serve as a valuable resource for individuals seeking to add healthy pounds. They aim not just to increase weight but to do so in a manner that prioritises overall health and well-being

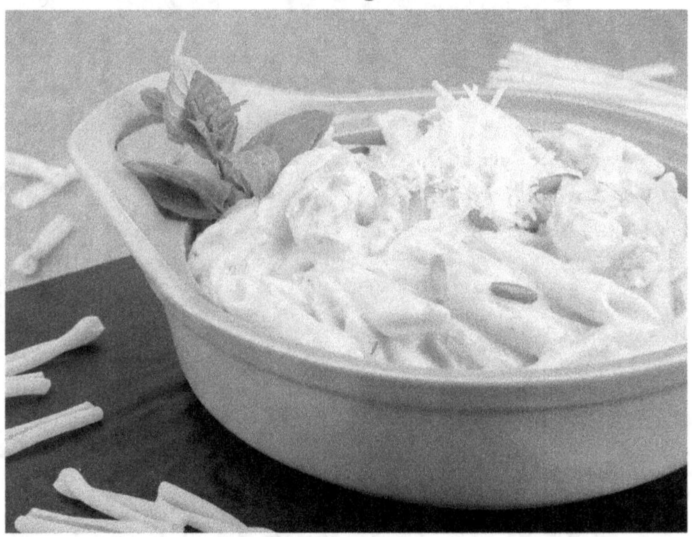

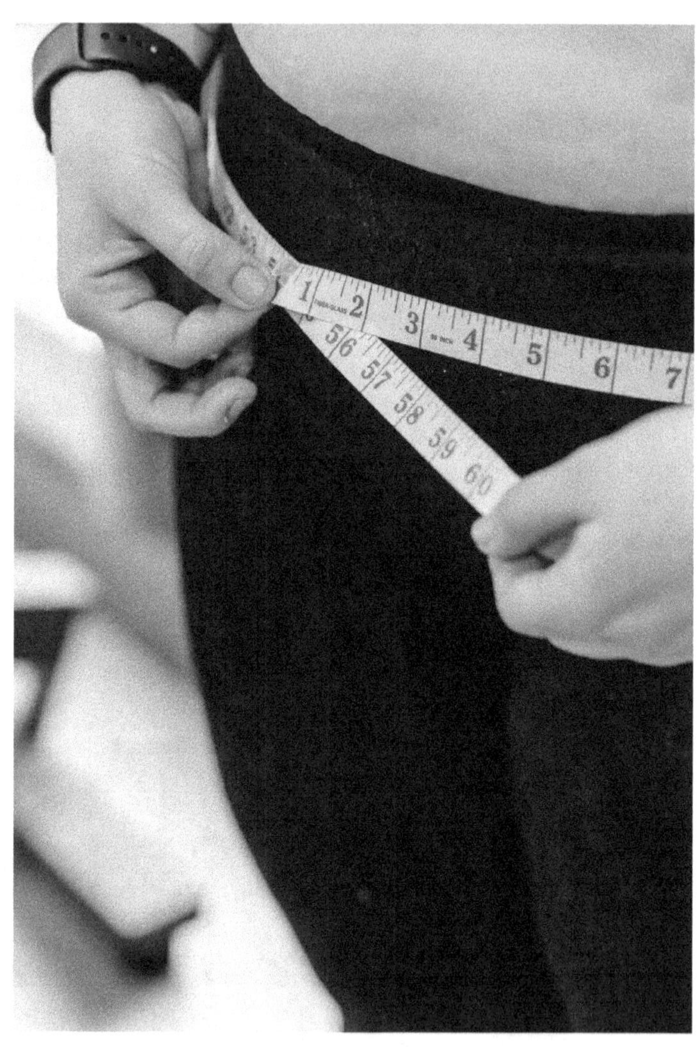

Chapter One

Breakfast Recipes

Breakfast serves as the foundation of a day's nutritional intake. For those aiming for weight gain, high-calorie breakfast recipes offer an excellent opportunity to kickstart the day with a substantial dose of nutrients and energy. These recipes focus on incorporating calorie-dense yet nutritious ingredients to support weight gain in a healthy manner.

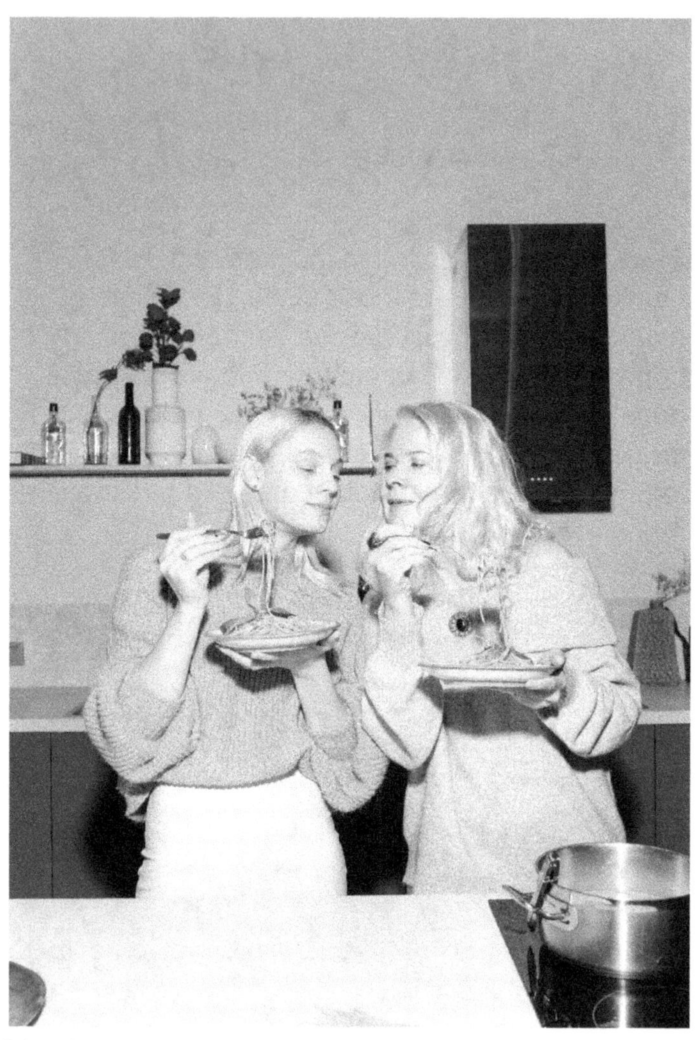

blend together a variety of ingredients such as bananas, oats, nut butter, Greek yoghourt, and protein powder. These concoctions provide a convenient way to pack in calories, proteins, and healthy fats in a quick and delicious manner.

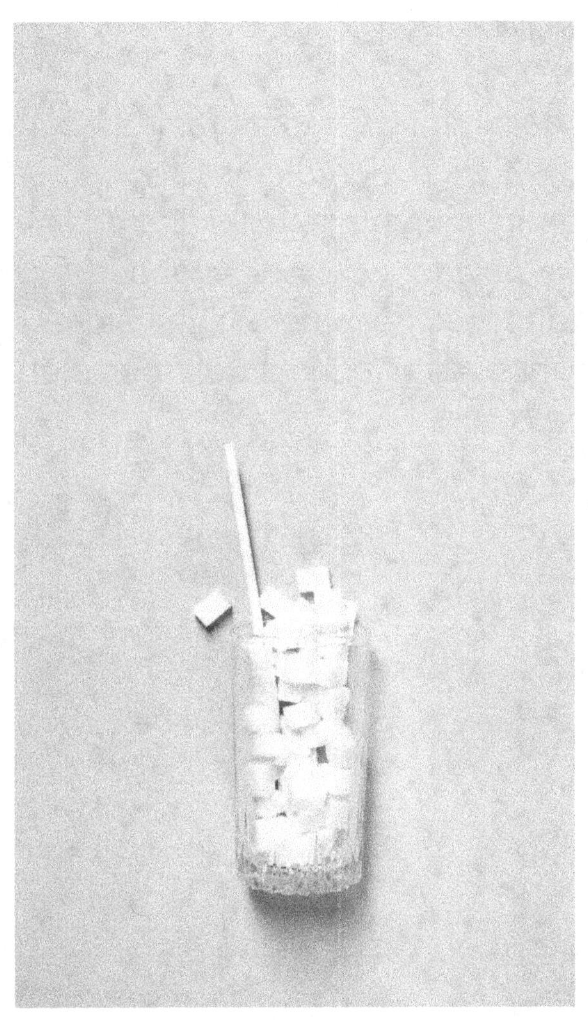

Protein-Packed Pancakes

offer a delightful twist to a breakfast classic. By using ingredients like whole-grain flour, eggs, milk, and adding in protein powder or Greek yoghourt, these pancakes become a high-calorie option while still offering a delicious start to the day.

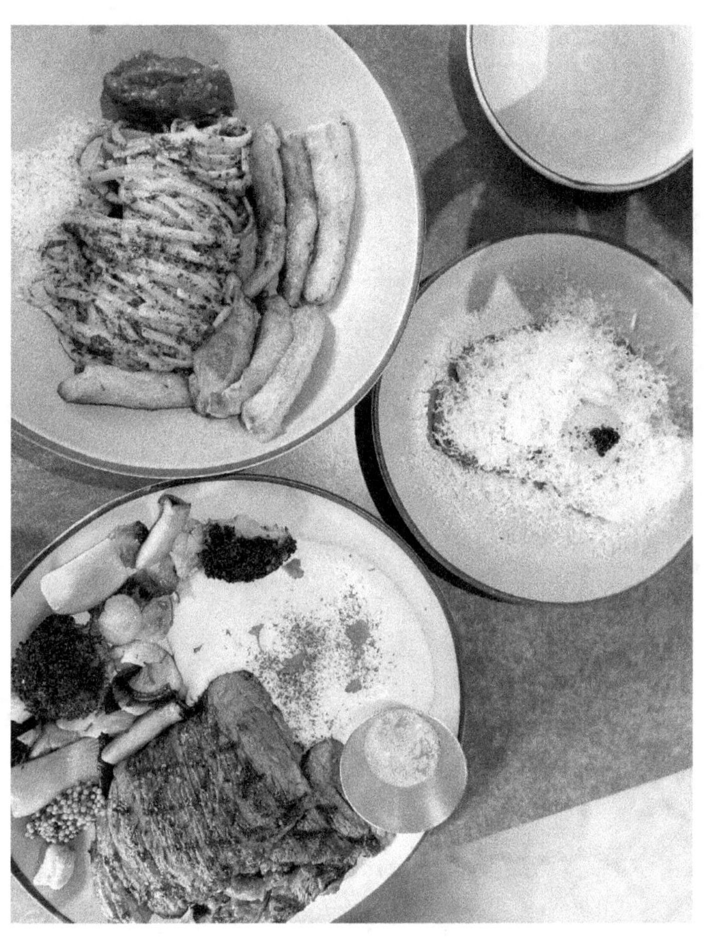

Nut Butter Toast Varieties

combine whole-grain bread with generous
spreads of almond, peanut, or cashew butter.
Topped with sliced fruits, seeds, or honey,
these toasts not only provide a calorie boost
but also offer a mix of healthy fats, proteins,
and carbohydrates for a balanced breakfast.
These breakfast recipes set the tone for a day
filled with energy and nutritional balance,
essential for those seeking to gain weight
healthily.

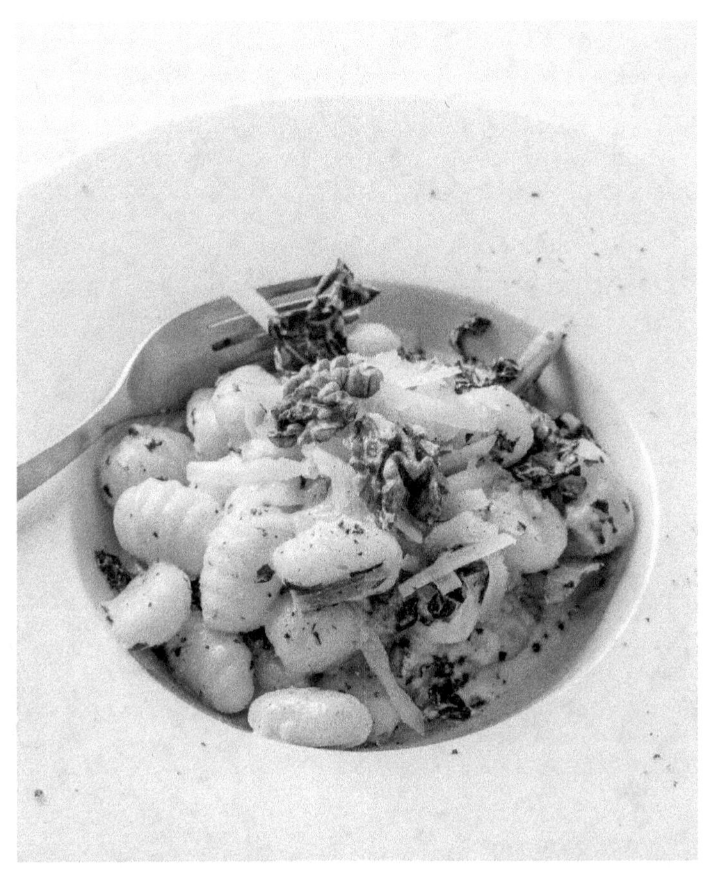

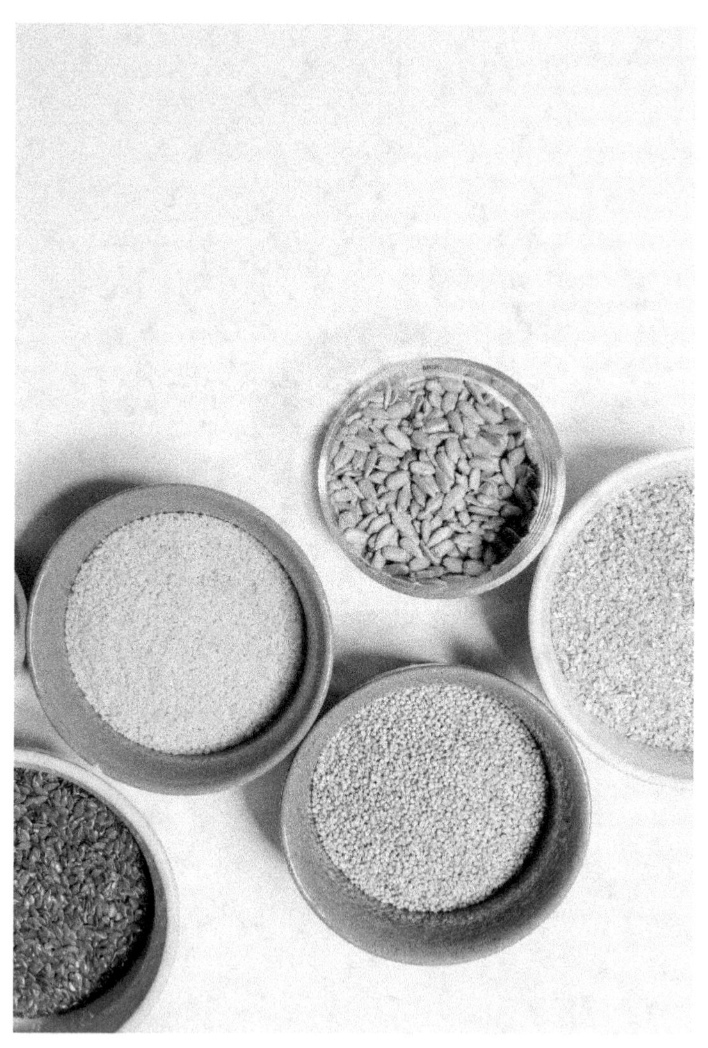

Chapter Two

Lunch and Dinner Options

Lunch and dinner present ample opportunities to incorporate calorie-dense, nutrient-rich ingredients into meals tailored for weight gain. These meals should strike a balance between providing a high calorie count and delivering essential nutrients necessary for overall health and well-being.

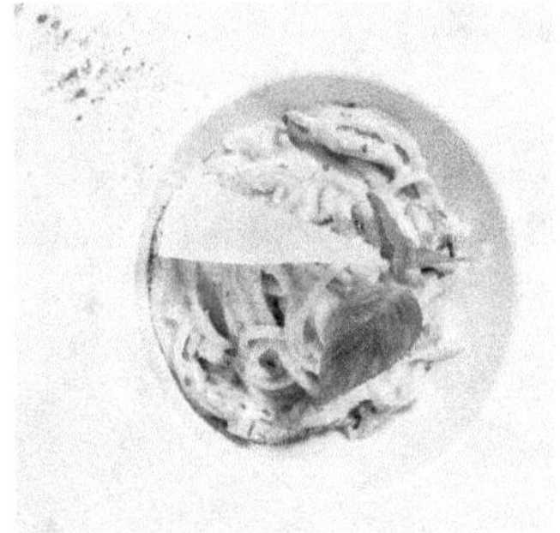

Creamy Pasta Dishes

form a versatile canvas for high-calorie recipes. By incorporating whole-grain pasta and pairing it with creamy sauces made from ingredients like cheese, cream, or nut-based sauces, these dishes offer a calorie-packed meal. Adding protein sources such as grilled chicken, shrimp, or tofu boosts the nutritional value while increasing calorie intake.

become a convenient lunch or dinner option. Wraps stuffed with rice, beans, cheese, avocado, grilled meats or plant-based alternatives, and a variety of vegetables offer a high-calorie punch. Adding guacamole, sour cream, or a drizzle of sauce further enhances both flavour and calorie content.

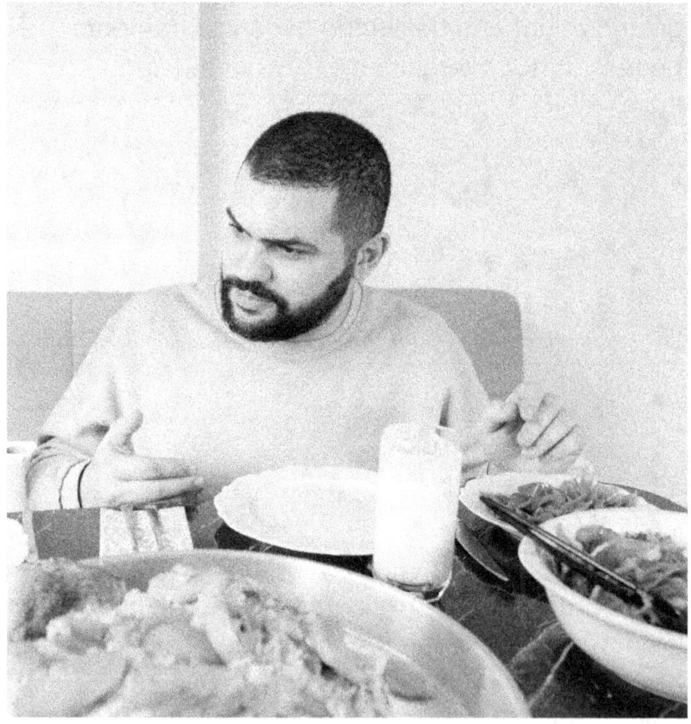

Cheesy Baked Casseroles

provide a hearty and satisfying dinner option. Combining layers of ingredients such as pasta, rice, vegetables, meats or plant-based proteins, and a generous amount of cheese creates a calorie-rich meal. These casseroles can be customised to include various ingredients while ensuring a substantial calorie intake.

These lunch and dinner options showcase the flexibility and diversity of high-calorie recipes for weight gain. They emphasise the inclusion of wholesome ingredients rich in calories, proteins, healthy fats, and complex carbohydrates to support a balanced diet aimed at increasing weight in a healthy manner.

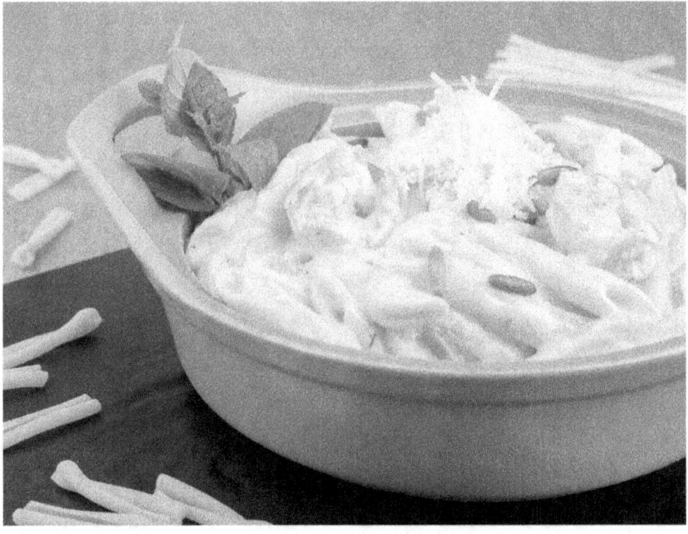

Moreover, these recipes offer room for customization based on dietary preferences or restrictions. For vegetarians or vegans, replacing meats with plant-based proteins like tofu, tempeh, or legumes ensures adequate protein intake. Similarly, individuals with gluten sensitivities can opt for gluten-free grains or pasta alternatives.

Incorporating a variety of colourful vegetables not only adds nutritional value but also enhances the overall taste and texture of these meals. Vegetables such as spinach, bell peppers, broccoli, and carrots not only contribute vitamins and minerals but also complement the richness of these dishes.

Furthermore, the cooking methods used in these recipes can also impact their caloric content. While baking, grilling, or roasting maintain the nutritional integrity of the ingredients, using healthy oils or fats for cooking can contribute additional calories. For instance, using olive oil, coconut oil, or avocado oil in meal preparation can increase the overall calorie count without compromising healthfulness.

In summary, lunch and dinner options for weight gain should focus on incorporating nutrient-dense ingredients in calorie-rich combinations. By customising recipes to accommodate dietary preferences and utilising various cooking methods and ingredients, individuals can craft meals that support healthy weight gain while ensuring a well-rounded nutritional intake.

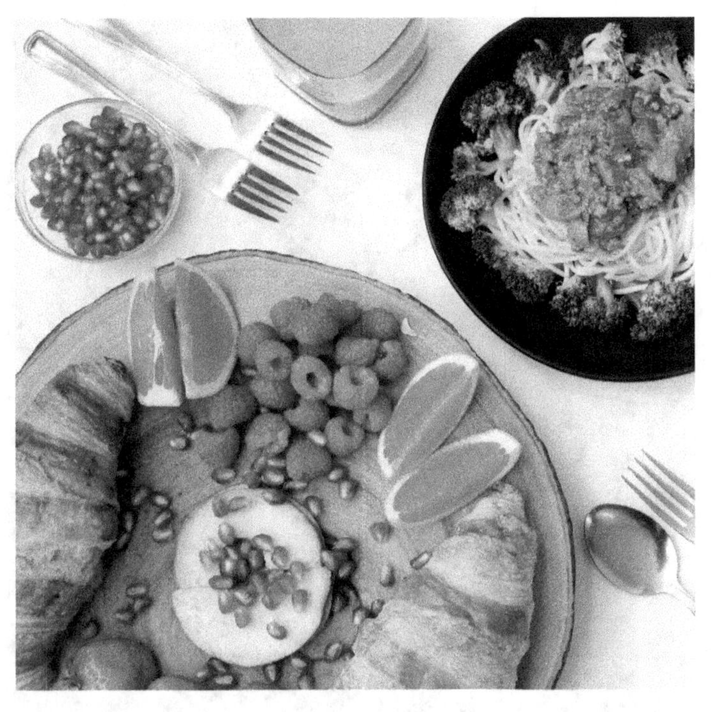

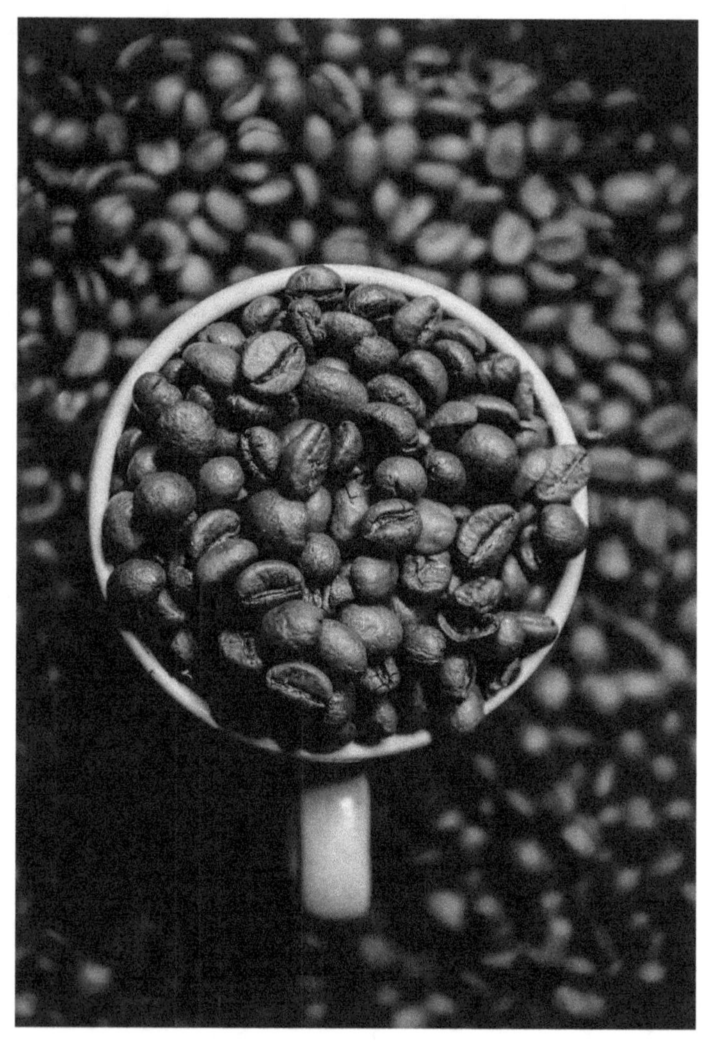

Chapter Three

Snacks and Small Meals

Snacks and small meals play a pivotal role in achieving weight gain goals by providing additional opportunities to boost daily calorie intake. Crafting high-calorie snacks requires a careful selection of ingredients that offer both nutritional value and energy-dense content. These smaller meals should complement the main meals, ensuring a consistent and balanced approach to calorie consumption.

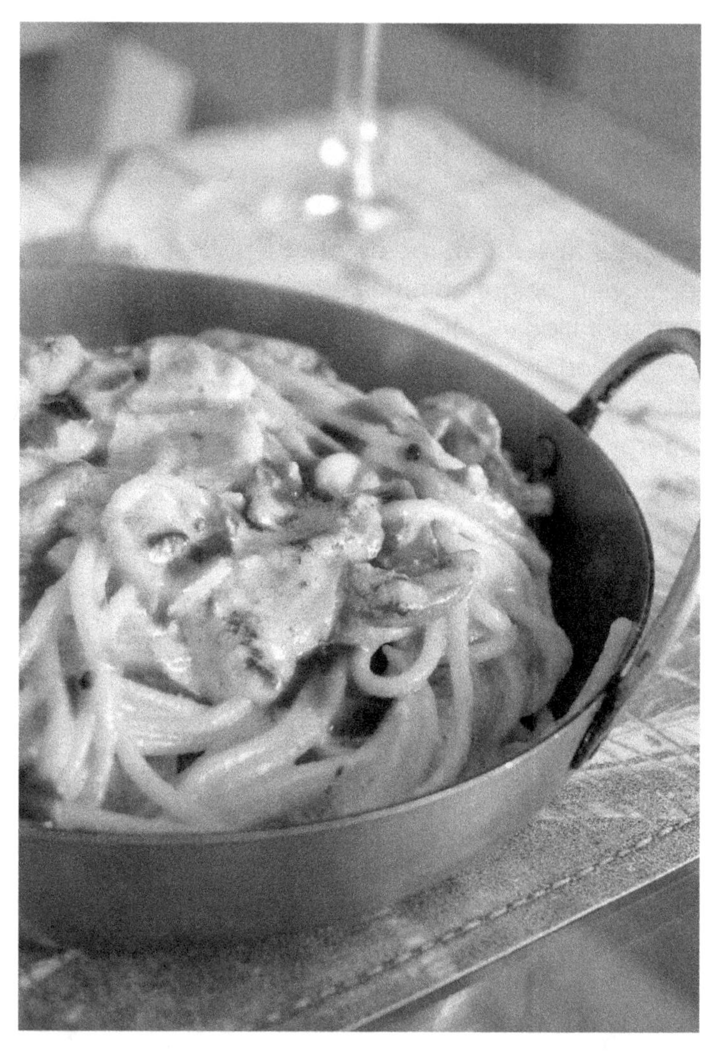

Energy-Packed Trail Mixes

stand out as a versatile and convenient snack option. Combining nuts, seeds, dried fruits, and even a sprinkle of chocolate or yoghurt-covered pieces creates a calorie-dense mix. Nuts like almonds, cashews, and walnuts, along with seeds like pumpkin or sunflower seeds, contribute healthy fats, proteins, and additional nutrients, making trail mixes an ideal on-the-go snack.

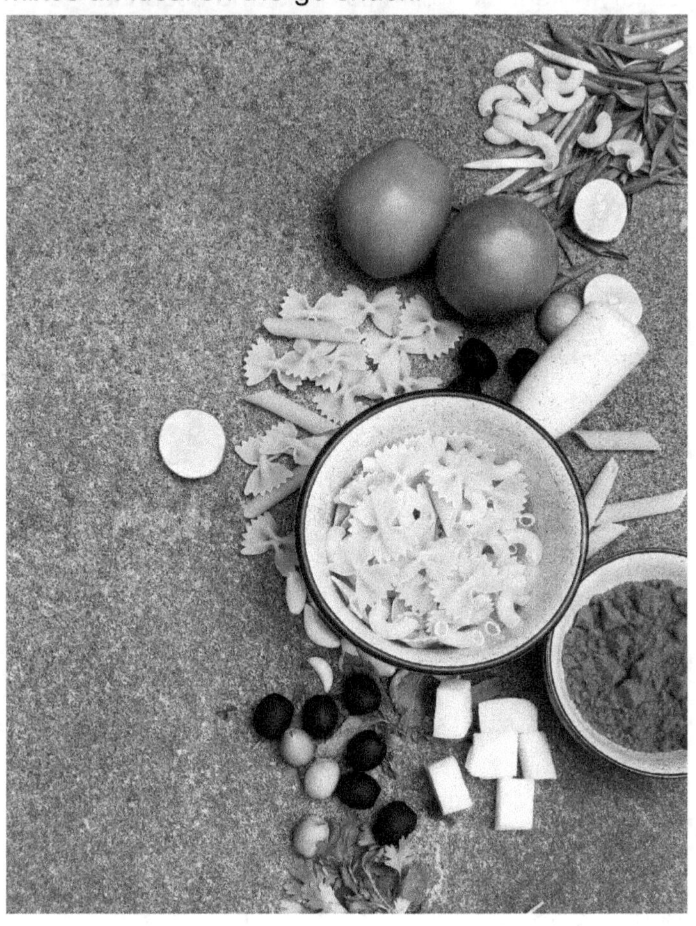

present a powerhouse of healthy fats and nutrients. Avocado slices on whole-grain crackers or mashed avocado spread on toast with toppings such as eggs, smoked salmon, or tomatoes offer a satisfying snack rich in calories and essential nutrients.

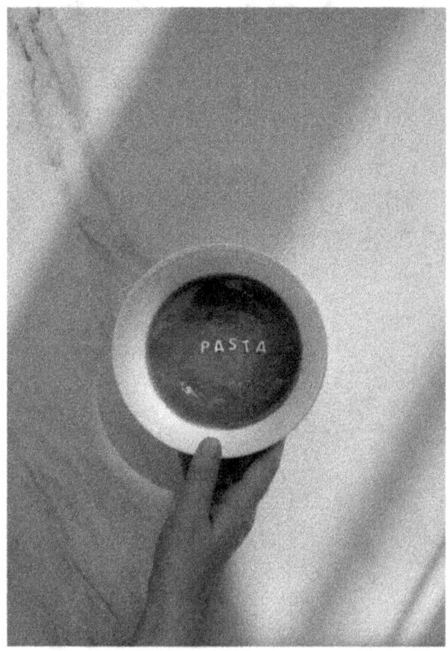

 provide a customizable option for a high-calorie snack. Combining oats, nuts, seeds, dried fruits, honey or nut butter, and even dark chocolate or coconut flakes allows for a nutrient-dense and calorie-rich snack bar. These bars can be tailored to individual taste preferences while ensuring a healthy balance of macronutrients.

These snack and small meal options are designed to bridge the gap between main meals, offering an additional calorie boost while providing essential nutrients. They are particularly beneficial for those seeking weight gain, as they aid in maintaining a consistent calorie intake throughout the day.

Moreover, these snack options can be adapted to suit various dietary preferences and restrictions. For individuals following a vegan or vegetarian diet, omitting animal products and focusing on plant-based sources of protein and fats can be easily incorporated into these snacks. Similarly, those with gluten sensitivities can opt for gluten-free variations of ingredients.

Portion control and frequency of consumption play vital roles in incorporating these snacks into a weight gain regimen. Eating smaller meals and snacks at regular intervals throughout the day helps in steadily increasing overall calorie intake without overwhelming the digestive system.
In addition to their high-calorie content, these snacks offer a blend of essential nutrients crucial for overall health. They contain a mix of vitamins, minerals, antioxidants, and fibre, contributing to a balanced diet essential for healthy weight gain.

Furthermore, preparing these snacks at home allows for better control over ingredients, ensuring they are free from additives, preservatives, or excessive sugars often found in store-bought alternatives. This not only enhances their nutritional value but also allows for customization according to individual taste preferences and dietary requirements.

In essence, incorporating high-calorie snacks and small meals into one's daily routine aids in achieving weight gain goals by providing additional nutrients and energy between main meals. These snacks serve as an integral part of a well-rounded dietary approach, emphasising both calorie density and nutritional value.

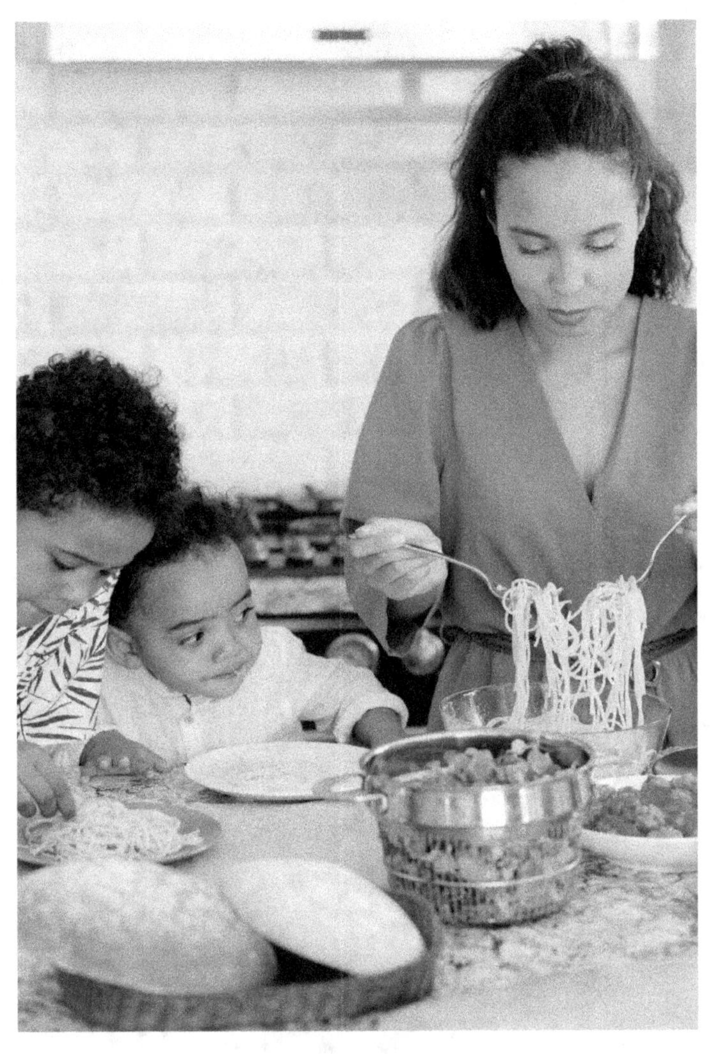

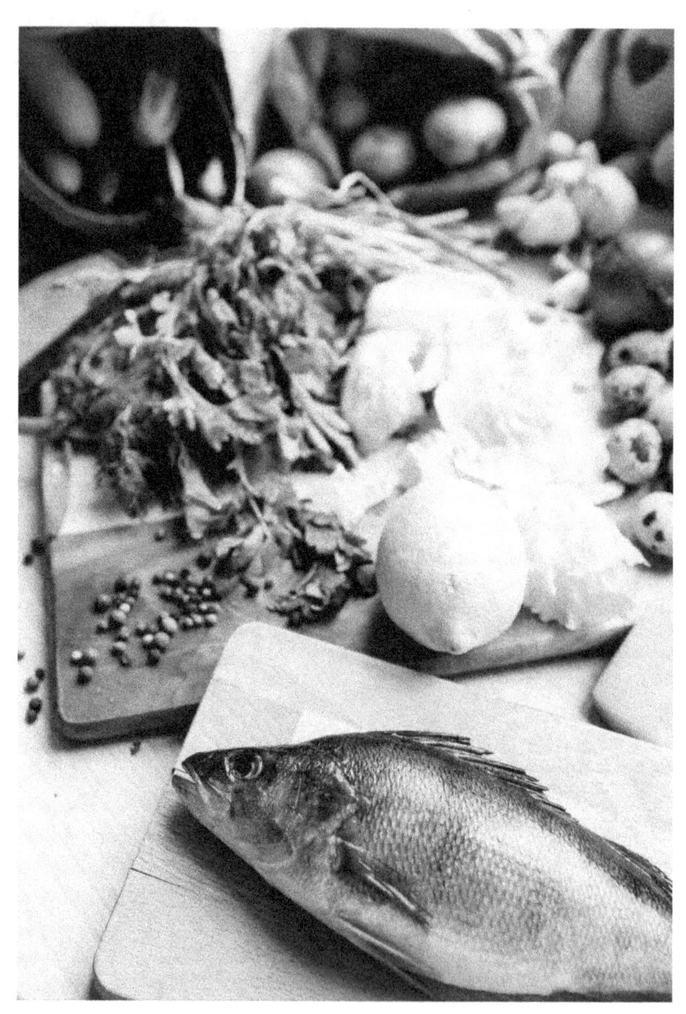

Chapter Four

Desserts and Treats

Desserts and treats serve as a delightful yet effective way to increase calorie intake for those aiming for weight gain. These recipes focus on incorporating calorie-dense ingredients while ensuring a delectable indulgence. While the goal is to boost calorie consumption, these desserts and treats aim to strike a balance between nutritional value and deliciousness.

Decadent Milkshakes

stand out as a calorie-rich dessert option. Blending together ingredients like whole milk, bananas, nut butters, Greek yoghurt, or ice cream creates a creamy and satisfying treat. Adding extras like chocolate syrup, caramel, or nuts further boosts the calorie content while enhancing flavour.

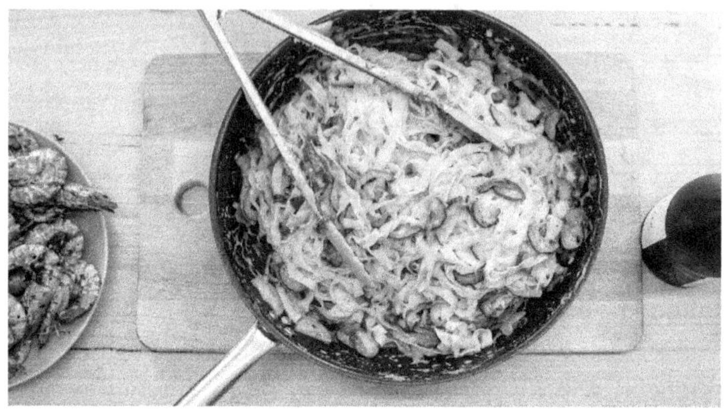

Rich Chocolate Brownies

offer a delightful way to indulge in a high-calorie dessert. Recipes that include ingredients such as butter, eggs, dark chocolate, nuts, and even additional mix-ins like caramel, peanut butter, or marshmallows provide a dense and calorie-packed treat.

High-Calorie Fruit Parfaits

offer a healthier yet equally satisfying dessert option. Layering Greek yoghourts with granola, nuts, seeds, and a variety of fresh or dried fruits creates a visually appealing and nutrient-dense dessert. Adding honey or a drizzle of chocolate sauce elevates the calorie count without compromising on taste.

are crafted to provide a significant calorie boost while offering a delightful conclusion to a meal. They incorporate ingredients that contribute to the overall calorie intake without sacrificing taste or nutritional value.

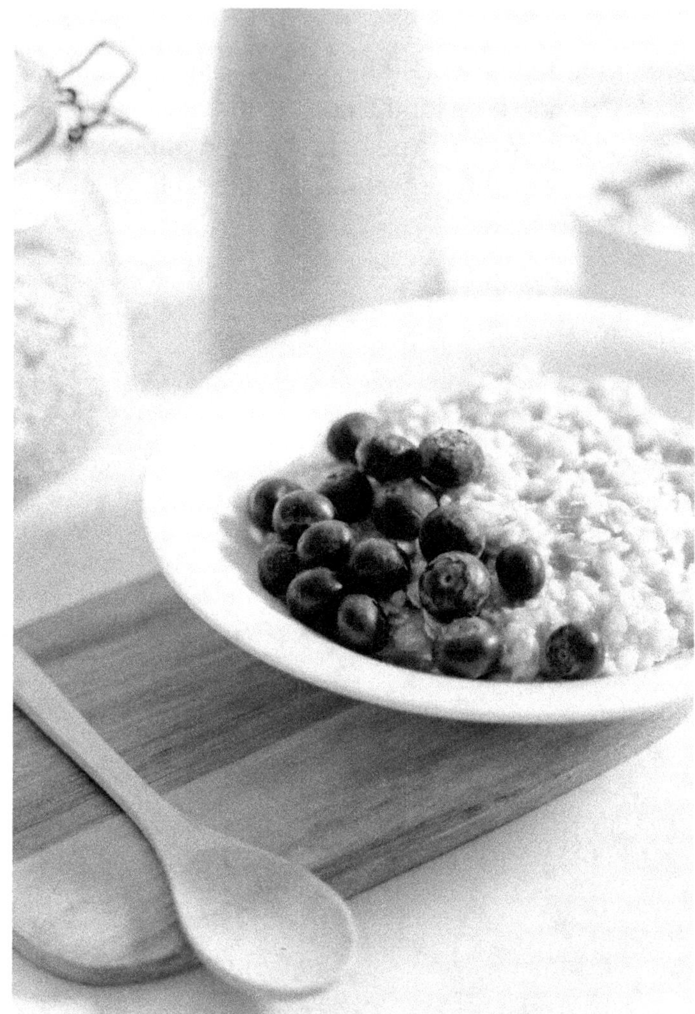

Furthermore, these dessert recipes allow for customization to suit different dietary preferences and restrictions. For those following a vegan or dairy-free diet, substitutions like plant-based milk, dairy-free chocolate, or egg substitutes can be used without compromising the overall richness of the desert.

Portion control remains crucial when incorporating these high-calorie desserts into a weight gain regimen. While they offer a delicious way to increase calorie intake, moderation is key to prevent excessive consumption of sugars and fats.

Apart from their calorie density, these desserts and treats can also provide essential nutrients. For instance, dark chocolate used in brownies or fruits in parfaits contribute antioxidants and vitamins, adding a layer of nutritional value to these indulgent treats.

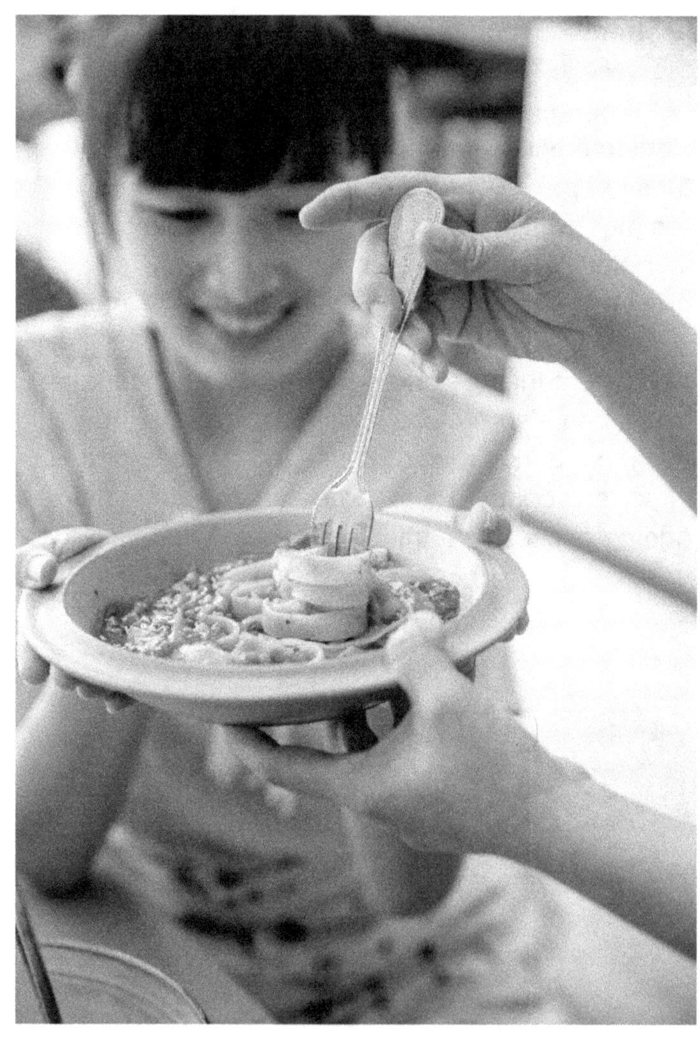

Preparing these desserts at home allows for better control over the quality and quantity of ingredients used. This ensures that these treats are free from artificial additives or excessive sugars often found in commercially available desserts. Homemade variations also allow for creativity and customization, tailoring the desserts to suit individual taste preferences and dietary needs.

In summary, desserts and treats designed for weight gain offer a sweet and satisfying way to increase calorie intake. They combine calorie-dense ingredients with delicious flavours, ensuring a balanced approach between indulgence and nutritional value. When consumed in moderation, these desserts become an enjoyable addition to a well-rounded dietary plan aimed at healthy weight gain.

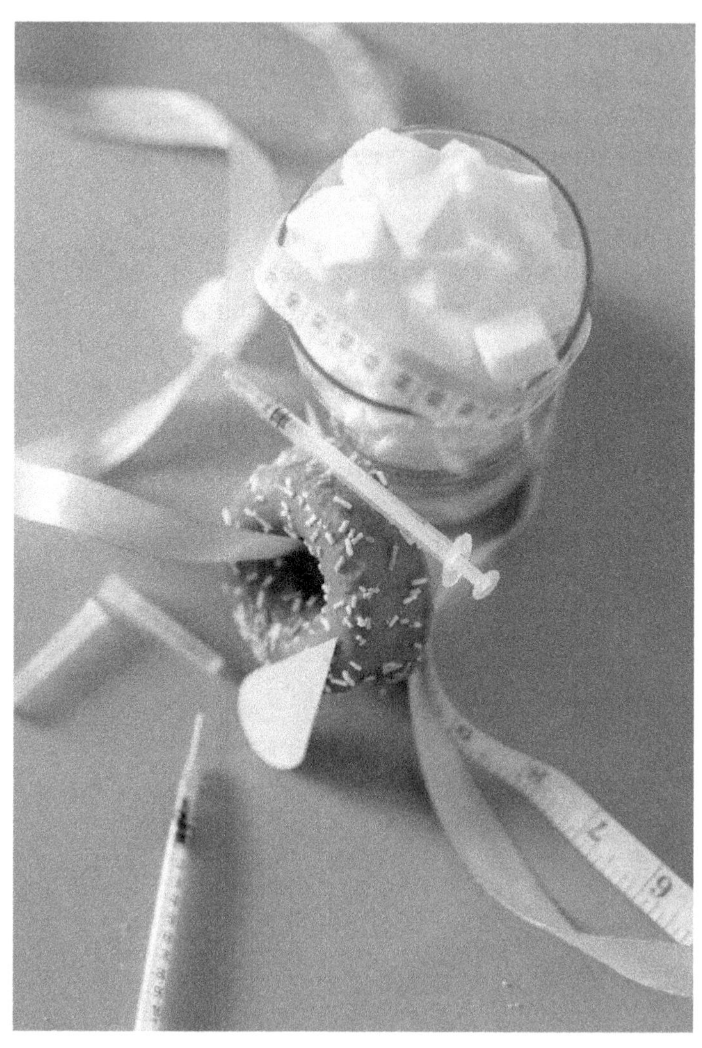

Summary

Calorie-Rich Creations: Nourishing Recipes for Healthy Weight Gain"

In a world fixated on weight loss, the quest for healthy weight gain often remains overlooked. "Calorie-Rich Creations" unveils a treasure trove of delicious, high-calorie recipes meticulously crafted to support healthy weight gain in a nutritious and balanced manner.

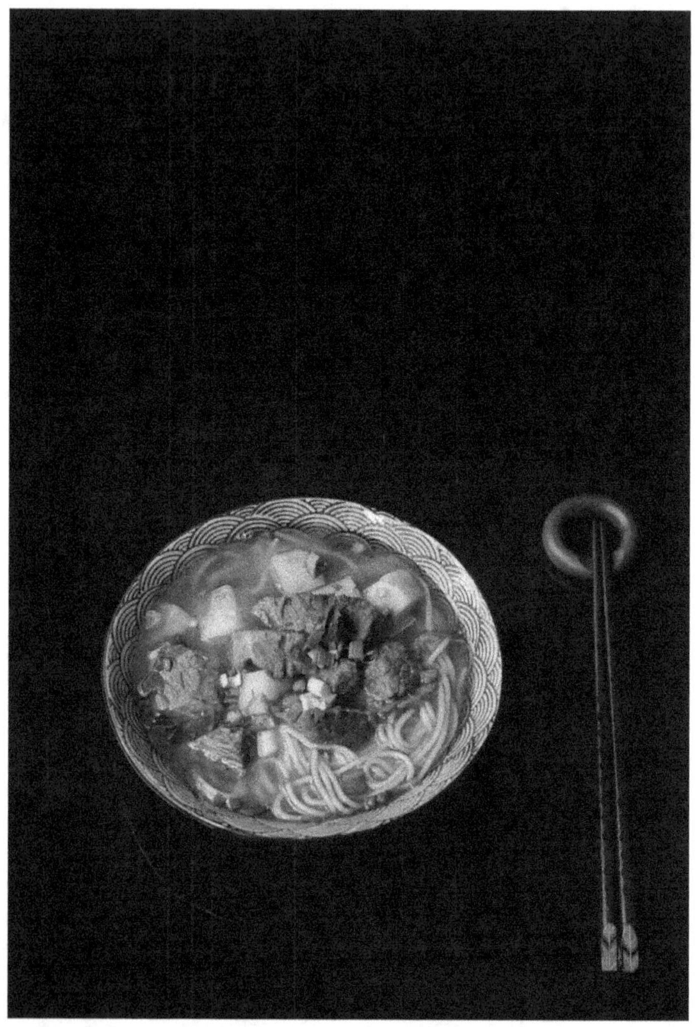

Dive into a culinary journey designed to empower individuals seeking to add healthy pounds or muscle mass. This comprehensive guide demystifies the art of increasing calorie intake through a repertoire of mouthwatering recipes, each meticulously curated to strike a delicate balance between indulgence and nutritional value.

Explore a wide array of meal options spanning breakfasts, lunches, dinners, snacks, and delectable desserts. From protein-packed pancakes at sunrise to creamy pasta dishes for lunch, and from energy-packed trail mixes for midday munchies to rich chocolate brownies for an indulgent treat, this book offers a diverse range of recipes tailored to suit different tastes and dietary needs.

Calorie-Rich Creations" isn't just a cookbook; it's a holistic guide that emphasises the importance of balanced macronutrients and micronutrients. Discover the significance of nutrient-dense ingredients like whole grains, lean proteins, healthy fats, and colourful fruits and vegetables in each meticulously crafted recipe.

This book is more than just a collection of recipes; it's a comprehensive resource featuring insightful tips,

suggested meal plans, and guidance on portion control, ensuring a practical and sustainable approach to healthy weight gain. With adaptable recipes accommodating vegetarian, vegan, and gluten-free preferences, "Calorie-Rich Creations" becomes an indispensable companion for anyone seeking a healthier path to increasing their weight in a mindful and nourishing manner.

Embrace the journey toward a balanced and thriving body with "Calorie-Rich Creations," where deliciousness meets nutritional wisdom in every delectable bite.

Conclusion

In the pursuit of weight gain, high-calorie recipes serve as a valuable tool for individuals seeking to achieve their goals in a healthy and balanced manner. These recipes offer a structured approach towards increasing calorie intake while emphasising the importance of nutritional value and overall well-being.

The fundamental principle behind high-calorie recipes for weight gain is to strike a balance between calorie density and nutrient richness. Each recipe incorporates a thoughtful selection of ingredients that contribute to a substantial increase in caloric intake while providing essential macronutrients (carbohydrates, proteins, and fats) and micronutrients (vitamins, minerals, and antioxidants). This balance is crucial in promoting healthy weight gain by ensuring that the additional calories consumed contribute to overall health rather than solely increasing body mass.

Moreover, these recipes are adaptable and versatile, accommodating various dietary preferences, restrictions, and lifestyle choices. Whether one follows a vegetarian, vegan, gluten-free, or other specialised diets, these recipes can be tailored accordingly, ensuring inclusivity and accessibility.

The practicality and accessibility
These high-calorie recipes make them feasible for everyday use. They offer simplicity in preparation, utilising readily available ingredients and straightforward cooking methods. This accessibility encourages consistency in incorporating these recipes into one's daily routine, thereby facilitating a steady increase in calorie intake.

It's crucial to understand that while the primary focus of these recipes is to boost calorie consumption, moderation and portion control remain key principles. Overconsumption of high-calorie foods, even when aimed at weight gain, can lead to undesirable health consequences. Therefore, these recipes should be integrated sensibly into a well-balanced diet, complementing main meals while preventing excessive intake of unhealthy fats, sugars, or processed foods.

Furthermore, the incorporation of high-calorie recipes isn't limited to the context of weight gain alone. These recipes offer a diverse array of nutrient-dense options that can benefit athletes, individuals recovering from illness, or those with higher metabolic needs.

Preparing these recipes at home allows individuals to take charge of their nutrition, ensuring that the meals are free from artificial additives or excessive sugars commonly found in processed foods.

Homemade variations provide the opportunity for customization according to taste preferences, dietary needs, and health goals.

In conclusion, high-calorie recipes for weight gain offer a comprehensive approach to achieving healthy and intentional weight increase. By emphasising nutrient density, balance, adaptability, and moderation, these recipes become a valuable resource in promoting not just weight gain but overall health and well-being. When integrated sensibly into a balanced diet and lifestyle, these recipes pave the way for a healthier and more empowered approach towards achieving weight goals.

Keywords

• Nutrient-dense recipes for weight gain

• Calorie-rich meal plans

• High-calorie foods for healthy weight increase

• Balanced macronutrients in weight gain recipes

• Customizable high-calorie diet plans

• Protein-packed recipes for muscle gain

• Wholesome high-calorie snacks and desserts

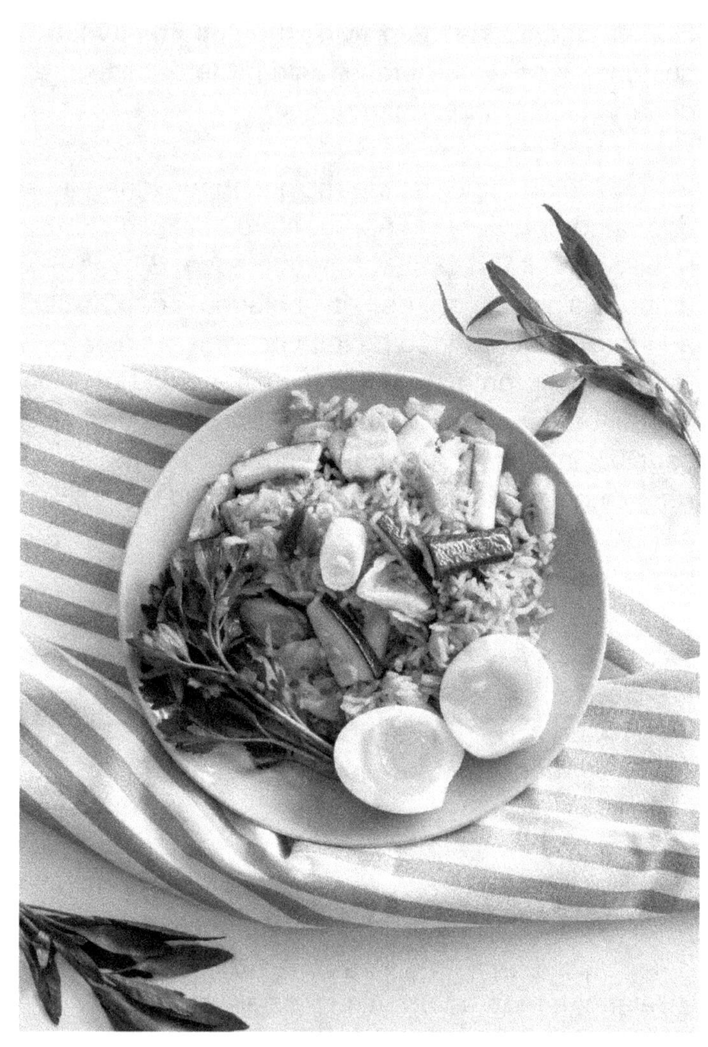

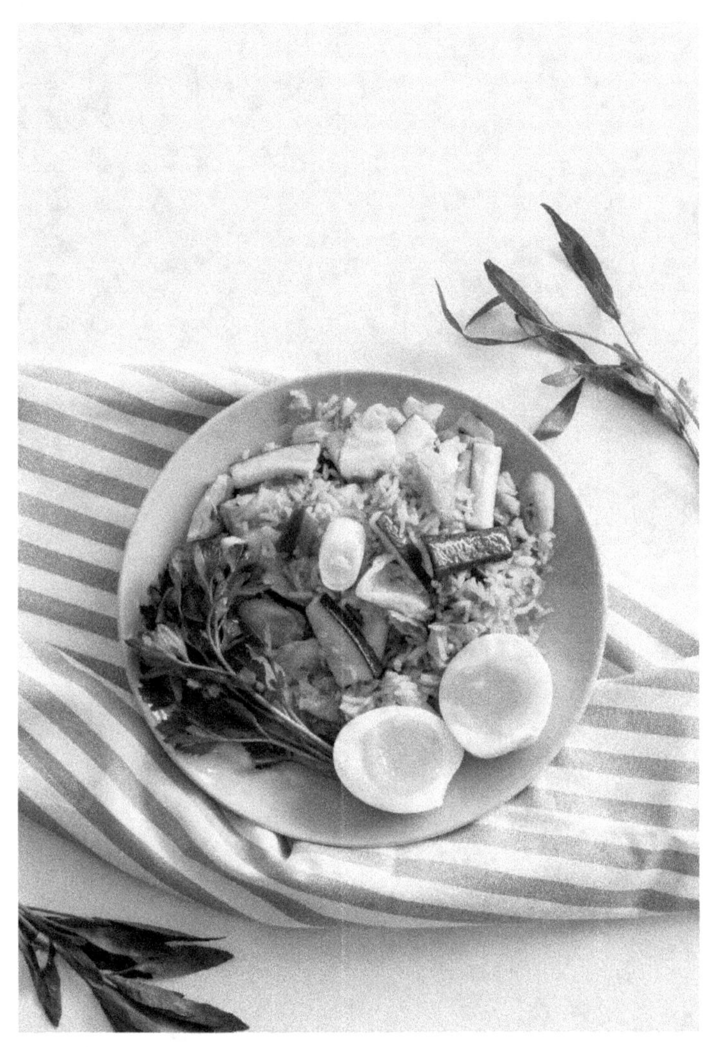